The
Gift
of
Cancer

*Miracles happen when you change your
thoughts and release the fear!*

Linda Ranalli-Marr

BALBOA
PRESS

A DIVISION OF HAY HOUSE

Balboa Press books may be ordered through booksellers or by contacting:

Balboa Press
A Division of Hay House
1663 Liberty Drive
Bloomington, IN 47403
www.balboapress.com
1 (877) 407-4847

Because of the dynamic nature of the Internet, any web addresses or links contained in this book may have changed since publication and may no longer be valid. The views expressed in this work are solely those of the author and do not necessarily reflect the views of the publisher, and the publisher hereby disclaims any responsibility for them.

The author of this book does not dispense medical advice or prescribe the use of any technique as a form of treatment for physical, emotional, or medical problems without the advice of a physician, either directly or indirectly. The intent of the author is only to offer information of a general nature to help you in your quest for emotional and spiritual well-being. In the event you use any of the information in this book for yourself, which is your constitutional right, the author and the publisher assume no responsibility for your actions.

Any people depicted in stock imagery provided by Thinkstock are models, and such images are being used for illustrative purposes only. Certain stock imagery © Thinkstock.

Print information available on the last page.

ISBN: 978-1-5043-6258-0 (sc)
ISBN: 978-1-5043-6278-8 (e)

Library of Congress Control Number: 2016911708

Balboa Press rev. date: 07/26/2016

For my precious son, Nate

Introduction

"I thought you were on anti-depressants."

"Pardon me?" I asked.

"You acted so happy at that time. I honestly thought you were taking something."

What my dear friend was saying was what I know many of my friends and family members were thinking: Linda is holding it up so well. She must be so scared inside. She is trying to be so positive on the outside, but surely she must be terrified on the inside. After all, her cancer wasn't caught early. A nine-by-eight-centimeter breast tumor was by no means small. How could anyone with that diagnosis be happy? How could anyone with that diagnosis, who was also raising a three-year-old child, be happy? Surely, Linda is putting on a great performance!

What most people didn't realize was that I *was* truly happy. My cancer experience was the best event in my life next to the birth of my son. How could it not be? What I learned and am about to share in this book is how I realized that I was in control of my life, including the cancer.

Immediately after I received the cancer diagnosis, I instinctively knew it was *my mind* that needed healing, and I also knew that I better figure out how to heal that mind quickly so that my physical body could begin to heal too.

But what I didn't realize at that time was how God was about to show me how.

Chapter 1

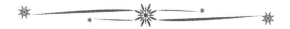

Life before Cancer

"What we are today comes from our thoughts of yesterday, and our present thoughts build our life of tomorrow: our life is the creation of our mind."

—The Dhammapada

I experienced a happy childhood. I grew up with an Italian Catholic background in a small town in Ontario, Canada. I attended university in Toronto and am now a kindergarten teacher.

As I reflect back, it was soon after my father's death from cancer, when I was twenty-one years old, that I began to be fearful of the "big C." Immediately after his passing, I began researching foods that contributed to the onset of cancer. I soon gave up red meat, followed by all meat years later. This decision was difficult for my Italian mother to accept since she took great pride in cooking authentic meat-based Italian dinners. In my twenties, I began conducting self-breast examinations on a monthly basis. When I would feel something abnormal, I would make an appointment with my doctor and wait to receive reassurance that I was fine.

When I turned thirty, I insisted on having a mammogram. Although my doctor didn't feel it was necessary at this age, I felt it was. I remember reading somewhere that it was a good idea to have a picture of your younger breasts as a reference in case I needed a breast comparison down the road.

As I grew older, my fear of getting cancer continued to grow. I began to avoid foods that came in any contact with chemicals. If I couldn't find organic fruits, I would make sure I peeled their skin. I would really scrub the skin on my vegetables in hopes of washing off all pesticides. I avoided the use of my microwave and cordless phones. I would only use laundry and dish detergent made from natural sources. Before my teaching career, I worked at a casino, and each day I would insist on working on the nonsmoking floor to avoid inhaling second-hand smoke. I remember getting into a heated discussion with the casino's general manager about the unhealthy working conditions he was allowing his employees to work under. Needless to say, he was not at all impressed by my opinion, and I soon learned to keep my thoughts to myself if I wanted to continue working there.

My mother would often tell me that I was acting in the same manner as my father. As I reflect back, she was right. Soon after my father's brother passed away from cancer, my father became fearful of the disease as well. I remember my father becoming a health fanatic soon after. He would begin shopping at health food stores and only purchased all-natural health care products. He cut down on eating red meat and often advised me to do so as well. He began exercising and eating plenty of fruits and vegetables, and he cut back on sugary foods. I remember my dad bragging about how youthful he looked due to his lifestyle changes, but I remember his fear as well. When I was thirteen years old, I remember my dad visiting various doctors whenever he suspected there was something wrong with him. When I would ask my mother about his visits, she would always say that he wanted to make sure he didn't have cancer.

My father and I shared the same fear. We both had a loved one die from cancer and automatically felt that we must be next. From where did this fear originate?

Many experts believe that cancer runs in the family, that there is a genetic component, but I now believe it runs much deeper than that. Soon after my diagnosis, I was shocked to listen to countless stories of people sharing with me how scared they were of getting cancer as well. One friend even said that her doctor stated that it wasn't a matter of *if* someone would get cancer but *when*.

Why this great fear? Can we place partial blame on a society that is bombarding us with endless stories that foster fear-based thinking?

There have been countless studies suggesting, in short, that *everything* gives you cancer. Outside the cancer facility where I received my cancer treatments hung a banner that read, "One in three people will get cancer." Imagine the fear-based thoughts this message is sending not only to the commuters who walk or drive by this banner each day but also to the cancer patients and their families. Imagine the thoughts that would be elicited from a banner that read, "More people are living healthier and longer lives than ever before." This fact is true. However, it is rarely given as much publicity.

In addition to being consumed by fear-based thoughts, I also used to lack a sense of joy. I had wonderful family and friends, but I was simply going through the motions. I was very fortunate to have gone back to work half time after my son turned one year of age. In many people's eyes, I had a perfect life. I taught in the morning and was home with my son by 12:30 p.m. He would take his nap, and I would often take one as well. I would have the rest of the day playing with my son. This was so ideal! However, I wasn't feeling the joy. Although my son's love was indescribable, I neglected myself. My main objective was meeting all of my family's physical and emotional needs, and at the end of the day, that didn't leave any time for me. I was simply going through life's motions, ignoring any opportunity for self-nurturance and attention. I didn't even bother to take notice of the awkwardness of my right breast while nursing my son, something I would have been on top of years earlier.

Chapter 2

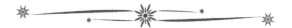

"Within each of us is a spark. Call it a divine spark if you will, but it is there and can light the way to health. There are no incurable diseases, only incurable people."

—Bernie Siegel, M.D.

I decided it was time to make an appointment for my physical examination. I hadn't had one since my son was born almost three years earlier. I remember being very consistent with my yearly physicals and self-breast examinations prior to having my son. I decided it was time to get back on track.

During my physical exam, my doctor felt a lump but wasn't very concerned because I was young (forty years old) and my breasts had always been lumpy and dense. My physician scheduled a mammogram just in case and told me that she would contact me only if there were any concerns. A few months passed, and I felt good that I hadn't received a phone call; I assumed my breasts were fine. However, I recall a conversation I had with a neighbor about her cancer experience. She stated that her mammogram didn't detect her tumor but an ultrasound did. This conversation motivated me to call my doctor to arrange an ultrasound appointment.

I was advised to pick up my mammogram report so that the ultrasound technician could refer to it. When I picked up and read the report, it stated that the findings suggested changes of sclerosing adenosis. Since I wasn't familiar with this term, I did on online search and saw that it said that if you had this condition, you also had a 50 percent chance of developing cancer.

Needless to say, I was shocked. My doctor never mentioned this to me. In the meantime, an ultrasound was taken on my right breast. I met with my doctor to discuss the results. My doctor was pleased to inform me that the results indicated I had two cysts located beside each other and that was the cause of the lump. I was happy to hear the good news. At this time, I handed her my mammogram report and shared with her the information I had researched. She stated that if I wished, she could schedule an appointment with a surgeon so a biopsy could be performed. My appointment was scheduled approximately seven months after the initial lump was found.

The first appointment with the surgeon was the worst day of my life. I knew from the surgeon's facial expression after she examined my breast that I had breast cancer. At this stage, my breast was revealing outward symptoms, such as dimpled puffiness on the edge of my breast. The surgeon was asking me various questions about my breast, all suggesting to me that she felt it was cancer too. She stated that she would schedule another mammogram, this time a magnified, close-up picture of my breast. I was told to return in two weeks. As she handed me the envelope to take with me to the hospital facility where I was to have my test, I read the following words: "Breast cancer suspected."

As I reflect back, it was clear that the next two weeks would be the worst two weeks of my entire cancer experience. In my gut, I suspected that I had breast cancer. However, in case I had any doubts, I was provided with explicit miraculous "signs" indicating I did.

I arrived home from my appointment and was relieved that I was by myself. My husband was at work, and my son was at the babysitter's. I was trembling inside. I needed to know. I needed to know if I had cancer. There was only one action that I knew I needed to do immediately to get my answer.

Be still, I told myself. I walked into my bedroom and sat up on my bed. I closed my eyes and took a few deep breaths. I was amazed that even during this most difficult time of my life, I felt a sense of peace. It was as if this warm feeling wrapped itself around me and whispered, *You will be all right*. As I sat there in stillness, I knew I would receive my answer. At this point I asked my higher power, "Do I have cancer?" My eyes were closed, and I only saw blackness. Not knowing what to expect, I suddenly saw in bright white capitalized letters the word *Yes*. I had no doubt at this moment that this was the truth. I was saddened by that moment, yet somehow I continued to feel a sense of peace. I thought to myself, *If cancer is what I have, then somehow, I'm not alone with it.*

This warm feeling continued to wrap itself around me, reassuring me that I would endure this journey with this protective presence by my side. It was this feeling of security and protection and love that I turned to throughout my journey. Whenever the fear would creep in, it was through being still that I was able to access this feeling of peace and knowingness. For me, I was able to access this feeling simply by crawling into my bed, sitting upwards, and becoming still with my thoughts.

During this time period, while waiting for the results of my mammogram, I immersed myself in books and magazines in order to distract my attention away from reality for a few moments each day. Although deep down I knew I had cancer, a part of me held onto the hope that I didn't. I oddly felt that if I distracted myself from my reality, then maybe what I was going through would turn out to be just a bad dream. Reading was one of those things that did that for me.

I began receiving a magazine subscription of Oprah's *O* magazine. The May 2010 issue arrived in the mail, and I was excited to finally enjoy a few minutes where my thoughts were not focused on cancer, or so I thought. I began skimming the pages of the magazine and came across an article titled, "The Big C: Customization," which focused on developing personalized cancer treatments. I was so disappointed to receive a reminder of what it was I was trying to distract myself from. With high hopes of distraction, I continued on until the next article caught my attention. My heart was flooded with disappointment. The following article titled, "The Truth is There," was about the journey of a woman with breast cancer. I was so saddened not only to have my attention directed toward cancer again, but by the intention of these articles. I instinctively knew my higher power wanted me to stop distracting myself from the possibility of not having cancer and directing me to the reality of having it. God was telling me to let go of this hope I was clinging onto. Still, even with these two cancer articles and God flashing the word *yes* across my mind, I still didn't want to believe I could have cancer. At this moment, I was prompted to do what I always did in the past when in need of a spiritual answer from God. I closed my magazine on my lap and asked my higher power to allow me to open up the magazine to a page that would give me the truth. My fingers opened up the magazine to an advertisement from the Breast Cancer Research Foundation. My heart sank. I was devastated. My hope of being healthy was gone.

This sign from God was the beginning of many spiritual signs that would lead me on the path of enlightenment and healing. From this moment on, God was going to provide me with an endless supply of miraculous signs all leading me to the direction of self-discovery. Through the specific asking, openness of receiving, I discovered a force within me that I never knew existed. It was this power that provided me with not only with the acceptance of the disease but the recognition of its blessing as well.

Chapter 3

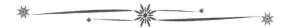

"If you think you can or think you can't, you're probably right."
—Henry Ford

Two days before my son's third birthday, I received a telephone message informing me that the results of my biopsy were in and that I needed to call the doctor for the results. I was happily surprised to receive this message. Surely, the doctor wouldn't be telling me bad news over the phone. She would call to set up an appointment if she was to reveal to me that I had breast cancer. But what about the spiritual signs that revealed to me that I had cancer? Could I have been mistaken about these signs? Was I reading too much into them? Were they just a coincidence? As much as I wanted to avoid making this phone call, I knew it was time.

The first thing the doctor asked me was, "Are you at home?" Thinking back to that question, what would the doctor have done if I weren't at home? What if I had been calling from a break at work and would have to return back to my classroom after receiving such devastating news? When I replied back that I was at home, the doctor proceeded to tell me that I had breast cancer. She said that due to the large size of the tumor, I would have to start with chemotherapy immediately, followed by surgery, and then radiation. She explained I needed to see an oncologist immediately in order to arrange my chemotherapy in hopes of preventing the spread of the cancer.

While struggling to process all this devastating information at one time, I somehow managed to ask the doctor a surprising question. "Tell me something positive." I remembered the long pause on the phone. She repeated the question to me and then found an answer. "You are young, and younger people tend to do better." Perfect, I thought to myself. I had something going for me at that moment, and I was going to run with it.

As I reflect back at that moment, I now see the huge shift I unconsciously decided to undertake when I asked that question. Despite the fact that I was just informed that I had cancer, the tumor was a huge size; I should be worried about it spreading, I would need to undergo chemotherapy within a few days, and I would begin to suffer all the side effects that come with it within the next few weeks, I decided to ignore these devastating facts and focus my attention and energy on one small advantage: my age.

As I hung up the phone and sat on my couch, I was embodied with a strong, intuitive feeling that it was *my mind* I needed to focus on in order to heal. It was my dysfunctional thoughts that had contributed to this disease in my body, and if I wanted to survive, I needed to figure out how to come to peace with these thoughts. Despite the fact that for the past twenty years, I had researched and attempted to do everything I could to avoid getting cancer from outside factors, somehow, I seemed to understand that it was my thoughts that I needed to heal in order for me to become cancer free.

At this point in my life, I not only had a great fear of getting cancer, but my mind was also entertaining negative thought patterns such as resentment, hatred, unworthiness, and feelings of helplessness. I had unsuccessfully attempted to heal those destructive thought patterns in the past. I was clueless on how to bring peace to my thoughts. I hated feeling this way, but I didn't have a clue on how to rid myself of it. Somehow, when I received the cancer diagnosis, there was a part of me that felt a sense of relief.

In a way, I felt that this cancer diagnosis was going to *force* me to heal these negative thoughts that were making my life unhappy. I knew that I was going to have to put a lot of time and energy into figuring out how to rid myself of these thoughts. This knowingness brought me a sense of peace. Once I figured it out and began to repair these thought patterns, not only would my body begin to heal, but I also would be happy again.

At that moment, I made the vital connection between the *mind* and the *body*. As a result, it was my number-one priority to figure out how to heal my "dis-ease" and begin the journey toward enlightenment.

Chapter 4

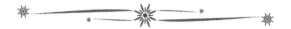

"When fear disappears, the foundation of disease is gone."
—Mary Baker Eddy

Soon after my diagnosis, the June 2010 issue of Oprah's *O* magazine arrived. I was hesitant to read this issue. I couldn't shake the feeling of disappointment and sadness that I felt while reading the previous issue. I didn't think I could bear to read another article about cancer. I had received enough disappointing signs.

I convinced myself that I would only briefly glimpse at the cover page. As I walked through the door with the magazine, I noticed a feeling of joy and happiness storm through me as I read the words, "Say Yes To Life." Tears began to fall. I instinctively knew its message! I needed to *choose* to say *yes* to my life. God was giving me this choice, and I had the power to accept it. I would survive if I *chose* to survive. I was overjoyed with happiness. Despite the devastating signs I received during the past issue, I was relieved to receive a sign of survivorship. At this moment, I was no longer hesitant to open up the magazine.

I excitedly flipped through the pages. I joyfully came across an article titled, "Slipping Past Borders." The article was about a woman with stage-four breast cancer who, seventeen years ago, had been given two years to live when she was first diagnosed. Amazing!

I was provided with an article of a woman with a poor prognosis of breast cancer like myself, and she was still alive seventeen years later. Without a doubt in my mind, this article's message to me signaled survivorship.

This magazine's cover headline and cancer article were the first of many miraculous signs that would unexpectedly and consistently reveal to me the message of survivor throughout my entire cancer journey.

Chapter 5

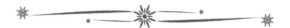

"If you think you have an incurable disease, if you think it yourself, you are right. If you think your problem is curable, then you are also right. It all depends on your intention (belief)."

—Herman Koning M.D.

Soon after receiving my June magazine issue, my husband and I visited with a local oncologist. Since my tumor was large, I was put on a priority list. Upon meeting the doctor, I was asked if I had undergone any additional tests to determine if my cancer had spread. I happily replied I did, and the results were negative. The doctor proceeded to tell me that the test results didn't carry much weight since the cancer could appear in my body later on. At that moment, I decided this was not the doctor I wanted treating me. If this physician was confident that I was going to get cancer down the road and wished to share her *belief* with me, then I was absolutely certain that she would not be chosen as my oncologist. As we left the office, I recalled stating to my husband, "She may not know it yet, but I'm going to be just fine."

As we arrived home, I was grateful to have received a telephone message with an appointment with another oncologist from a larger cancer facility approximately one hour from our home. Since I knew in my heart that I could not force myself to be treated by a doctor who shared her negative belief about my future health status, I was looking forward to meeting with a different oncologist the very next day.

While driving to that appointment, I kept repeating to myself over and over again, "This will be a positive appointment. This will be a positive appointment." When I finally met with the oncologist, I instantly knew from the warm smile she gave me as she walked into the room that I was going to feel comfortable and safe having this person as my oncologist. Near the end of the visit, the doctor had examined my breast, and I will always remember her surprised reaction as she examined me. She said that she had felt larger tumors than mine before. She was expecting to feel a larger tumor based on the results of my biopsy report. Wow! That's wonderful! My tumor wasn't the largest she has examined before. This was great news. I chose to focus on this!

As I reflect back on my reaction to this visit, I see how I unconsciously decided to once again focus on the one positive aspect of this visit: my tumor wasn't the largest this physician had seen. I could have easily chosen the fear-based thoughts and focused on the fact my biopsy result must be so serious that this physician expected to examine a tumor size that was larger than she had ever examined before.

Somehow, throughout my cancer journey, it wasn't difficult for me to approach my illness with a degree of optimism. Since I instinctively felt this was *a mind-based illness,* my job was to find a way to heal my thoughts while allowing the doctors to heal my body. At this point, I was redirecting my thoughts toward the one spiritual sign I had received thus far that signaled to me survivorship: the June 2010 issue of *O* magazine. When the fear-based thoughts began to creep in, I would pick up the magazine and read and reread, "Say Yes to Life." The knowingness of its message would crush instantly any fearful thoughts that would emerge. Peace would then settle in.

Chapter 6

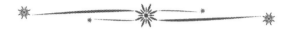

"There is no illness of the body apart from the mind."

—Socrates

It took me getting cancer to finally stop fearing it. I experienced twenty years of living my life fearing cancer, and now that I had the disease, I was experiencing a sense of relief. I saw how my dysfunctional thought patterns and resistant thoughts about getting cancer contributed to its development. Florence Scovel Shinn writes in her book, *The Florence Scovel Shinn Reader,* "When man is harmonious and happy, he is healthy! Resentment, ill-will, hate, fear, etc., tear down the cells of the body."

Louise Hay, author of *You Can Heal Your Life*, states that "There are really just two mental patterns that contribute to disease: fear and anger. Anger can show up as impatience, irritation, frustration, criticism, resentment or jealously. Fear could be anxiety, worry or unworthiness. When we release this burden, all the organs in our body begin to function properly."

I was *happy with cancer* because by fully owning up to my dysfunctional thoughts and seeing its relationship to my disease, I felt liberated in some way. Illness doesn't just occur at random. It's a by-product of our vibration and thoughts that we are generating. I felt *happy with cancer* because I was not only being driven to release my dysfunctional thought patterns, I was moved to direct my thoughts to one of healing and health instead.

I'm not suggesting that I never experienced fear. I believe roughly 20 percent of my thoughts were fear driven. The miracle was not the low number of fearful thoughts I experienced but what I attempted to do to stop it. I was well aware of the importance of stopping this fear in order to heal my body. *The Secret* author, Rhonda Byrne, states in, *The Secret Daily Teachings*, "When you are afraid of something happening, by the law you attract it, although fortunately it takes real focus and persistent fear to bring it to you. The amount of emotion you invest in not wanting something to happen is powerful. At the same time, it is also impossible to bring what you want when you hold so much fear about the outcome you don't want. Remove your personal investment of fear from what you don't want to happen and use that powerful energy and direct it to what you want. No matter what you have been thinking or feeling, your power to create something new is now."

I was happy with cancer because I now understood how my fearful thoughts of getting cancer, coupled with my dysfunctional thoughts of helplessness, hate, and unworthiness assisted in the development of the disease. I was happy with cancer because after learning that I had the power to attract this disease through my unhealthy thoughts than surely I possessed the power to heal my body of it as well. I was happy with cancer because after twenty years of fearing cancer, *I finally released it!*

Chapter 7

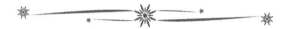

"The secret of health for both mind and body is not to mourn for the past, not to worry about the future, or not to anticipate troubles, but to live the present moment wisely and earnestly."
—Siddartha Guatama Buddha

When faced with a serious, life-threatening disease—especially with my poor prognosis—crushing the fear-based thoughts was not always easy. However, I used various strategies that I wish to share that would not only be useful in stopping the fear of cancer in your thoughts but in stopping any thoughts that are creating anxiety, stress, or tension within you.

First, whenever a fearful thought about cancer (or any dysfunctional thought) would emerge, whether it was thoughts of guilt, resentment, unworthiness, hate toward others, and so forth, in the beginning I would literally scream, "Stop!" During this one time period near the beginning of my treatments, I was experiencing hateful thoughts toward one particular person, and I was unsuccessful in my attempts at making peace. I had no idea how to stop thinking of this person in such a negative way.

I knew it was unhealthy for me to feel this hatred, but I lacked the knowledge I needed to stop it. One morning, I remembered taking a shower and watching as my long blonde hair was falling off and landing on the shower floor. As devastating as this experience was, I found myself shocked at how, during this saddened moment, I was thinking of this one particular person. *How is that possible?* This made me even more furious toward this person. *I'm losing my treasured hair, and all I could think about was this person. Insanity!*

Finally, I decided to do something about it. While in the shower, I decided to scream at the top of my lungs, "Stop!" while tears and hair fell down my body. I decided to scream a few more "Stops," each one with less volume than the previous. After I finished my shower, I shockingly discovered that when I yelled, "Stop!" my thoughts toward this person had actually stopped. A few minutes later, new thoughts toward this person would emerge, and I would repeat this process over and over again. Soon I began to softly say, "Stop," until the next thought, and then after a while, I would begin to say it quietly to myself.

What happened as a result of doing this repeatedly was life changing for me. Hateful thoughts toward this person began to diminish in frequency. By simply saying to myself, "Stop," each time a thought about this person emerged, the thoughts toward this person would appear less often in my mind. By intentionally stopping these thoughts from entering your mind, they lose their power over you.

I couldn't help but begin to feel great joy and peace knowing that I now had the control to stop these thoughts from entering into my mind space. With consistent practice, the thoughts begin to diminish until you begin to take notice of the peaceful space that is left in your mind.

This practice of screaming, yelling, or softly saying the word *stop* can be applied to any thoughts that are entering your mind uninvited.

I soon began using this technique whenever the fear of cancer would resurface. Whenever my mind or the voice in my head would try and convince me that I had a lot to fear, I would suddenly say, "Stop" to that voice.

One night, while reading a bedtime story to my son, the book featured a dinosaur character that refused to take his medicine. He would fling the medicine bottle into the air whenever his mother attempted to give him some. I instantly took a liking to the word *fling*. From that moment on, whenever a fear-based thought about cancer would appear, I would simply tell it to "fling." Whenever my mind felt the need to remind me of the size of the tumor, and I felt fear of reoccurrence, I would simply say, "Fling!" and the thought would vanish. Whenever I would sense people's fear of the disease, I would "fling" their fear so that I wouldn't be affected by their negative energy.

Simply put, whenever I would experience any type of fear-based thoughts that cancer patients experience on a minute-to-minute basis that robs them of the joy of living, I would simply "fling" it. Once again, with repeated practice, the ego-based thoughts of fearfulness begin to lose its power, and you begin to notice that the thoughts have diminished in frequency. Finally, you gradually begin to experience peace within your mind.

Eckhart Tolle, author of *A New Earth*, explains this mental process. "Notice the voice in the head, perhaps in the very moment it complains about something (fear) and recognize it for what it is: the voice of the ego, no more than a conditioned mind-pattern, a thought. Whenever you notice that voice, you will also realize that you are not the voice, but the one who is aware of it. In fact, you are the awareness that is aware of the voice. In the background, there is the awareness. In the foreground, there is the voice, the thinker. In this way you are becoming free of the ego, free of the unobserved mind. The moment you become aware of the ego in you, it is strictly speaking no longer the ego, but just an old, conditioned mind- pattern. Ego implies unawareness. Awareness and ego cannot coexist. The old mind-pattern or mental habit may still survive and reoccur for a while because it has the momentum of thousands of years of collective human unconsciousness behind it, but every time it is recognized, it is weakened."

Whenever the voice in my head (ego's voice) would attempt to scare me by thinking thoughts of cancer/fear, I would automatically identify those thoughts as "my ego." I would literally say, "That's my ego right now wanting me to be scared." As soon as I made this awareness, the fear-based voice loses its power and stops it in its tracks. As Eckhart Tolle stated, these thoughts will reoccur for a while, but the more you are "aware" of these thoughts and attribute them as "ego thoughts only," then they begin to not only lose its power, but they appear less often in your mind space because "awareness and ego cannot coexist."

I also believe that it is of upmost importance to begin teaching children how to identify ego based thoughts at an early age so that they may grow up not only being aware of their thought patterns but knowing they have control over them as well. Whenever my son is thinking thoughts that cause him unhappiness, he simply tells those thoughts to "Stop!" I have also shared with him how it is our "ego" that is telling us to think of things that cause us fear and unhappiness. How joyful it is to hear my son tell me whenever I am thinking aloud fear-based thoughts, "Mommy, it's your ego that is making you think that." Many of my friends have also shared this technique with their children and take delight in hearing their young ones tell their ego thoughts to "Fling" or "That's enough."

By taking control of your thoughts and eliminating the occurrence of negative based thoughts, you are leaving yourself open to thinking thoughts of creating your life the way you want to experience them. As author, Rhonda Byrne states in her book, *The Power*, "Sometimes your mind can take off like a freight train down a mountain without a driver, if you don't stay in control of it. You are the driver of your mind, so take charge and keep it busy with your instructions by telling it where you want it to go. Your mind only takes off on its own if you're not telling it what to do."

"The mind acts like an enemy for those who don't control it."
—Bhagavad Gita (Fifth century BC) ancient Hindu text

Chapter 8

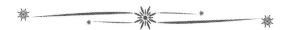

"People need to realize that their thoughts are more
primary than their genes, because the environment, which
is influenced by our thoughts, controls the genes."
—Bruce Lipton, Ph.D., American cell biologist

When I was learning how to control my fearful thoughts about cancer, in addition to focusing on my belief of surviving this disease, I had no idea that this was having a physiological effect on my body. I was just happy that my thoughts weren't focused on cancer every minute, and that I was able to experience peaceful thoughts during what could have been a very difficult time period in my life. By "flinging" my fearful thoughts, I was in fact activating my body's healing capacities.

Author and cell biologist Dr. Bruce Lipton asserts that you may be able to change how your DNA is expressed based on what you believe. When M.D. and author of *Mind Over Medicine,* Lissa Rankin, questioned him on how belief can change the cellular environment, Lipton explained, "The brain is perception, but the mind is interpretation. It's all about how the mind interprets a life event. For example, you can open your eyes and see a person (the perception), and your mind interprets this person as scary, the brain releases stress hormones and other fear chemicals that damage the cells. When we shift the mind's interpretation of illness from fear and danger to positive belief, the brain responds biochemically, the blood changes the body's cell culture and the cells change on a biological level. As it turns out, changing your thoughts can actually change how your brain communicates with the rest of your body, thereby alerting the body's biochemistry."

Lissa Rankin further states, "When our beliefs are hopeful and optimistic, the mind releases chemicals that put the body in a state of physiological rest, controlled primarily by the parasympathetic nervous system, and in this state of rest, the body's natural self-repair mechanisms are free to get to work fixing what's broken in the body. If, however, the mind thinks negative beliefs, the brain perceives these as a threat. As far as the brain is concerned, there's a lion running after you, so it's time to fight and flee. When the body's stress responses are activated, the body isn't concerned with long-term issues like cellular rejuvenation, self-repair and fighting the effects of aging. It's too busy preparing you to run away from the lion. No point putting your immune cells to work chewing up stray cancer cells or turning over fresh new cells in the body if you're about to get eaten. Over time, these negative beliefs that repetitively trigger the stress response take their toll. The cellular environment gets poisoned with stress hormones. It's no wonder the body gets sick and has a hard time repairing itself."

By learning how to control my fear-based thoughts of cancer as well as believing that as long as I could "Say yes to life," then my body was going to naturally begin the process of healing. This meant that my thoughts were actually having an impact on the approximately 70 trillion cells in my body!

Chapter 9

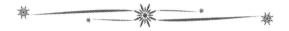

"Every happening great or small is a parable
whereby God speaks to us and the
Art of Life is to get the message."

—Author unknown

Not only was I successful in controlling my fear-based thoughts of cancer by telling them to "fling," I also learned to ask for and be open to receiving spiritual signs that would reassure me that I was going to survive this disease. Asking and receiving signs reinforced my belief that I was going to survive. Once again, this belief, combined with turning away from threatening thoughts, was having a positive impact on my physical body.

I am well aware that many people would regard this particular strategy as irrational, questionable, and perhaps unattainable. Let me reassure you that with an open mind, this strategy can be very powerful in not only controlling your fears and providing you with the gift of knowingness but also in allowing your body's innate healing powers to take over. When fear is lifted, the body can relax and focus on healing. Whenever I would receive a sign, I would experience this enormous feeling of relief take over me. I would feel my entire physical body just let loose and allow the fear and tension to melt away. Knowing now how the physical body can begin repairing itself once a threat or fear is lifted, I highly recommend this strategy to those who are open to receiving them. Receiving such signs to me was equivalent to God holding up a sign that read, "You will survive." I truly feel that God is delivering signs to us every day, and it is up to us to be open to receiving and reading these signs. Once he recognizes that you are receptive to receiving them, then he will deliver more. However, if you are continually dismissing them as a coincidence or regard them as foolishness, then the signs will not be plentiful.

Perhaps you are questioning whether it is God's intention for you to survive. Perhaps you think that maybe your time has come, and you are simply allowing what is meant to happen occur. If you begin asking for signs, perhaps you are afraid of receiving a sign that signals death. How do you know if this is what God wants for you?

You need to believe that we were not sent to this earth to suffer and experience sickness. We were sent here to experience joy and be the creators of our life. The reason you became ill was because there was a breakdown in your thinking patterns that created a disease. Your creator only wants you to be able to heal your thought patterns and your physical body so that you can begin to experience joy and creation again. You were given the healing power to heal your body the day you were born. Thus, God will only send you signs of survivorship because this is what *he wants from you*. This is why he has granted this power within you to heal. Your *belief* about his intention for you and your ability to heal is paramount to your survivorship.

The first step in receiving spiritual signs is to *ask*. Ask the universe, your higher power, or God for signs and be specific on your intention. For example, ask for a sign that when you see it you will immediately sense that the sign was meant for you. Ask for a sign that, when you receive it, you will automatically know it signals survivorship. Once you ask for a sign, release it to the universe and expect it to happen. Do not focus on it or fear that you will not receive it. This will delay its coming.

Florence Scovel Shinn has stated in her novel, *The Florence Scovel Shinn Reader,* that, "Man must make the first move. I have often been asked just how to make a demonstration (or request a sign) and I reply: Speak the word and then do not do anything until you get a definite lead. Demand the lead, saying, 'Infinite Spirit, reveal to me the way, let me know if there is anything for me to do.' The answer will come through intuition or hunch; a chance remark from someone, or a passage in a book, etc., etc."

I would further suggest that if at first you receive a sign and are experiencing difficulty in accepting it as yours, do not hesitate in asking for another sign until you feel certain it was meant for you. Furthermore, when you first take notice of a sign, it is natural to doubt its intention, attributing the sign to mere coincidence or simple craziness. Your intellectual mind begins to discredit it. After receiving hundreds of miraculous spiritual signs, I soon learned that you needed to really take notice of your first gut reaction of a sign within the first few seconds to really determine its meaning or message. Some people refer to this gut feeling as their sixth sense, an intuitive feeling or an instinct. Regardless of what you call it, it is that feeling you get when you just know something without really knowing how you know it. After your initial reaction, your reasoned mind begins to rationalize it, and in the process you lose its intended message. Always go back to that first intuitive reaction when in doubt.

Furthermore, when you notice a sign, be prepared to receive the message in various forms. For example, your message can be a passage from a book, a song lyric, a conversation with a friend, or a reoccurring symbol that keeps popping up. It can even be something very unique and personal that only you would take notice of it. Once again, it's the initial intuitive gut reaction that will signal to you its purpose and meaning. Once you are open to receiving them, a beautiful occurrence begins to happen: *you will begin to receive more.*

Chapter 10

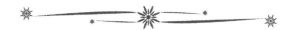

"The greatest miracle on Earth is the human body. It is
stronger and wiser than you may realize, and improving
its ability to self heal is within your control."
—Dr. Fabrizio Mancini

I consider myself very lucky that when I was diagnosed with cancer,
I was already receptive to receiving signs. I overcame the doubting
phase and was open to its gift. As a result, I began receiving signs about
my health status even before my doctor's phone call. Throughout my
cancer journey, I would receive numerous and various signs at those
moments when I needed them most; usually when the fear would
begin to creep in. The signs that I received were varied or repeated.
For instance, I would hear a song on the radio from either Sheryl
Crow or Melissa Etheridge; both breast cancer survivors. Usually, I
would hear them when I was experiencing fearful thoughts or while
I was driving and asking for a sign to bring me comfort.

I also would run into people I knew who were breast cancer
survivors—once again at the right moment I needed to receive it.
One of my favorite things to do when I needed an immediate sign
was to choose one of my spiritual books and ask my higher power
to have me open up the book to the page that I need to read for
whatever purpose. During the beginning of my illness, I was reading

Wayne Dyer's book, *Real Magic*, and after asking my higher power for spiritual guidance, I opened it to a passage that read, "Treat yourself as a well person and not allowing your mind to sabotage your body with the expectation of illness. Learn to act as if the miracle you seek in your mind is already here." Once again, peace and knowingness settled in.

I highly recommend recording these miraculous signs in a journal each time you receive them. This can be an excellent tool you can use whenever fear begins to creep in. You may assume that you will remember each one, but you would be surprised at how often we tend to forget. My journal was kept on my night table beside Oprah's June magazine issue. Whenever I would begin to experience fearful thoughts, I would walk into my room, sit on my bed, open my journal, and begin to read all the signs I received thus far that reassured me I would be fine. Sometimes, all it took was for me to walk into my room, glance over at the words, "Say Yes to Life," and turn around within seconds, leaving my room with the fear left behind me. To this day, I still refer to this practice whenever I visit my oncologist for my check-ups. I would reassure myself that my higher power had already told me through my signs that I was healthy and there was nothing to fear.

God has more knowledge about my body than a physician does. While waiting for my physician in the waiting room, I would simply go over in my mind all the signs I had received, and I begin to feel normal again. There is no greater reassurance that comes from knowing that your creator has supplied you with signs indicating that you will be okay.

Chapter 11

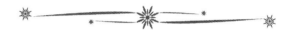

"We are taught that the imaging faculty plays a leading part in the game of life. What man images, sooner or later externalizes in his affairs. To play successfully the game of life, we must train the imaging faculty. A person with an imaging faculty trained to image only good, brings into his life every righteous desire of his heart – health, wealth, love, friends, perfect self-expression, his highest ideals."

—Florence Scovel Shinn

One of the most powerful spiritual signs that I received during my cancer journey that I still refer back to years later are Oprah's monthly *O* magazines. It was the magazine's articles that signaled to me, without a doubt, that I had cancer, and it was the subsequent articles that reassured me each month that I would survive it. These magazine articles that I received each month in the mail were incredibly and miraculously focused on the experiences I was going through during that particular month during my cancer journey. Having received many signs throughout my life, I remember being in awe each time as I opened up the magazine only to read an article in which the predominant message was specifically geared toward my fears or experiences that month. It was as if God was working through the magazine editor. I felt as if the editor knew my fears and experiences that particular month and decided to assign stories that would ultimately bring me the knowingness that I would survive. Even my skeptic husband, who would deliver my magazine to me each month, would sit quietly beside me as I read the magazine, waiting in anticipation for me to share in amazement its personalized message.

During my first month into chemotherapy, my girlfriend introduced me to the book, *The Secret* by Rhonda Byrne. The book discusses the method of attracting what you want through applying three steps: imagine it, feel it, and receive it. The book describes the first step as, "Use your mind to focus on and imagine what you desire. Imagine yourself *being* with your desire. Imagine yourself *having* your desire." It further described a tool you can use that can help you imagine your desire.

It recommends creating a vision board with cut-out pictures of the things you wish to receive. This was an easy concept to do because I clearly wanted to be healthy and live a long life, enjoying and engaging in various activities with my family. I immediately purchased a large corkboard picture frame and began cutting out pictures of the types of things I wished to do years down the road. I also posted pictures of myself before the illness so that I could look at pictures of myself in a healthy body. I made sure I placed it where I would see it several times a day. I would now recommend posting these pictures as well as inspiring messages or verses all over your house. It is suggested that by looking at the pictures each day, your desired thoughts will travel into your subconscious mind. Once a thought or belief is in your sub-consciousness, then this belief will manifest into reality.

Since this was the first time I even heard of the power of visualization, I was a bit sceptic. How could this simple concept of imaging what you want actually bring forth your desires, in particular, healing my body? Just as I was questioning this technique of visualizing what I wanted, I was provided with further signs pushing me toward this unfamiliar concept.

First, as I was flipping through old magazines looking for pictures for my vision board, I shockingly came across an article describing how to create your own vision board. The person creating the vision board in the magazine was my favorite Canadian musician, Jann Arden. I knew instinctively that God wanted me to take notice of this concept by including my favorite musical artist. I excitedly look over at her vision board, and I took note of one particular person she decided to attach to her board: Olivia Newton-John, who is also a breast cancer survivor.

The following sign was clearly directing me to take notice of this vision concept. It continues to bring me goose bumps whenever I think about it. One morning, I went to collect my mail at our community mailbox across the street, and I noticed someone had posted an advertisement on the side of the box. This was not an uncommon practice. Usually, there were people posting messages about a missing pet or used vehicle for sale. During this particular morning, I was drawn to read a newly posted message. What I read next sent chills up my body. There on my mailbox was a piece of paper that read, "Create your own Vision Board for 2010! Host your own Vision Boarding Enlightenment Party—three hours of fun, empowerment, and insight."

I simply stood there, unmoving for several moments, staring at this paper in disbelief. Having been accustomed to receiving hundreds of spiritual signs, this was the first time I stood still in complete shock. I quickly took notice of the only torn section of the paper where the contact number was located. At that moment, I decided to take a walk down the street to where the other two remaining neighborhood mailboxes were located. I've noticed on my walks that people tended to place their advertisements on these two mailboxes since they were relatively close to one another. Not surprisingly, both mailboxes are missing this flyer. I walked back to my mailbox and continued staring at it. I quickly grabbed the ad and placed it in my pocket. I knew that if I didn't, I would be questioning what I saw the very next day.

I knew at that moment, I had to begin envisioning my life as a healthy person without cancer. I had to imagine it *now!*

From that moment on, I attempted to imagine my body without cancer. I would picture the tumor in my mind and watch it as it left my body, floating upwards and disappearing through the top of my head, out of my body. When I went for my morning walks, I thanked God in advance for taking this cancer away. I would simply repeat over and over again each day for a few minutes, "Thank you God for taking cancer away from my body. Thank you God for taking cancer away from my body." Initially, I would simply repeat this without much feeling, but after a few weeks I found myself repeating it with some feeling attached to it. I was beginning to feel what it would be like if the tumor was *actually* removed from my body. I would feel elated, so I made sure to feel this way when I repeated the affirmation each day.

Apparently, many influential people and celebrities have credited a large part of their achievements to visualization, including Albert Einstein, Michael Jordan, Oprah Winfrey, Thomas Edison, and Arnold Schwarzenegger. Sports athletes would use this technique to prepare themselves mentally before a game or race. Tiger Woods has long used the power of his mind to form images and visualize exactly where he wants his golf ball to stop. When actor Jim Carrey was poor and living in a Volkswagen van, he would drive to the top of a hill overlooking the city of Los Angeles. It was there that he wrote himself a check for ten million dollars for "acting services rendered." He dated it three years later. When things got tough, he'd pull it out and look at it to remind himself of his dream. Just before the three years were up, he signed up to do *Dumb and Dumber* and was paid $10 million to play that role.

The goal of visualizing and repeating positive affirmations is to have that vision enter into your subconscious where your beliefs are stored. As Dr. Flavio Iammarino, Ph.D, states in his article, "How Do We Learn?" "The conscious mind gathers information and makes judgements, which it gives to the unconscious mind. The unconscious mind is designed to execute whatever we think. It is given information according to our random thoughts: both positive and negative. Regardless of whether the information is true or false, the unconscious mind creates a reality of whatever information it is given. In that way the unconscious mind is like a big room and the conscious mind is like the door to the big room. Whatever is allowed into the room is what will create a person's reality. Once we become aware of how our mind works, then we can consciously control our thoughts. And as we control our thoughts and repeat only good thoughts, we are becoming unconsciously competent. Now we have learned how to become far more powerful and we are able to overcome all stress and every fear. The unconscious mind is now able to go into autopilot and create every reality that we have intentionally planted into our lives using our thoughts."

I had no idea that by visualizing the tumor disappearing and repeatedly giving thanks for this, I was sending new messages into my unconsciousness. My unconscious mind was now receiving *new messages* about the cancer. It was now taking note of new cancer-free messages I was inputting. Knowing that the unconscious mind has no idea whether the information given is accurate or not, it begins to manifest into reality what new information it is now given.

By visualizing and repeating healthy affirmations on a daily basis, something magical started to happen. I started to *believe* that the tumor was gone. This became apparent on the day my surgeon called to book my surgery date for my mastectomy. When I hung up the phone, I recall sitting down on my couch and thinking to myself, "Why do I have to have surgery when I don't have cancer?"

After a few seconds, I remembered that indeed I did have cancer, and I needed to have it removed. While reflecting back, I was surprised at my initial reaction of actually believing the tumor had disappeared. Simply by repeating my affirmation and visualizing the tumor escaping my body during my morning walks, I actually began to change my belief toward the tumor's existence. Little did I know at that time, that *my vision's goal was actually becoming reality!*

I decided to open up my June issue of *O* magazine and finish reading the articles I missed. I opened it to an article titled, "The Vision Thing," describing how to create a vision board while envisioning your life the way you would like it to be.

"Imagination is the true magic carpet."
—Norman Vincent Peale (1898–1993)

Chapter 12

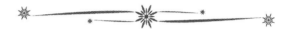

"Life expectancy would grow by leaps and bounds
if green vegetables smelled as good as bacon."

—Doug Larson

Soon into my cancer journey, I began receiving signs about foods that I should be eating and foods that I needed to omit from my diet. Immediately after my diagnosis, I began watching *Dr. Oz* and took notice of how many of his show topics were focusing around foods that kill cancer. I recall one particular episode where he had singer Sheryl Crow on discussing the foods she ate while undergoing breast cancer treatments. I carefully took note on what she was eating, not only because she had breast cancer, but also because many of my spiritual signs involved her. Many times when I would be driving and fear would creep in, I would ask God to deliver me a sign to remove this awful feeling. Sure enough, her songs would come on the radio. As a result, there wasn't a doubt that her appearance on *Dr. Oz* was not only intended to deliver me peace but also to direct my attention to foods that heal.

I immediately began eliminating all sugar, including natural sugar from fruit. I soon learned that sugar and red meat allowed cancer cells to grow. I was fortunate that I was a vegetarian and didn't need to worry about meat restrictions. I also eliminated all wheat products and dairy, except for eggs. By simply eliminating these foods, I surprisingly noticed the tumor shrinking considerably before the onset of chemotherapy. Since the tumor size was large, it was easy for me to feel the changes. The outer section of my breast where the tumor was located had developed outward physical changes. With the simple elimination of the above listed foods, these physical signs disappeared within weeks.

I also began learning about how certain foods were beneficial in attacking certain tumors as well. As a result, I filled my diet with lots of green vegetables, beans, nuts, certain spices such as turmeric and garlic, fish, and brown rice pasta. I also drank four cups of green tea each day. Not only did these food choices along with the chemotherapy work together in shrinking the tumor, but I experienced greater energy levels. I actually had more energy and felt healthier while eating these foods and undergoing chemotherapy than I did prior to my illness. I stopped taking naps with my son. With the exception of three days where my legs were sore due to the particular breast cancer chemotherapy drug, I never felt the need to rest. I was walking one hour each day as well as engaging in yard work such as cutting grass, creating new flower beds, digging dirt and so forth.

I do believe that it was a combination of things that delivered me with new energy levels during a time period where my body was being filled with poisonous injections. Clearly the new food choices as well as healing my dysfunctional thought patterns and relying on my spiritual signs to bring me comfort all worked together on renewing my energy levels.

When the July 2010 issue of *O* magazine was delivered, the artist featured on that month's article titled "Live Your Best Life" was none other than Sheryl Crow.

Chapter 13

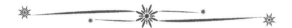

"To enjoy good health, to bring true happiness to one's
family, to bring peace to all, one must first discipline
and control one's own mind. If a man can control his
mind he can find the way to Enlightenment, and all
wisdom and virtue will naturally come to him."

—Buddha

It was now two months into my cancer journey, and I had just
finished chemotherapy and was awaiting my surgery. At this point,
I was feeling great physically and spiritually. I felt that I had received
plenty of spiritual signs that signaled to me that I was going to be
fine. However, there was a new fear that began to emerge in my
thoughts: the fear of reoccurrence. Although I was confident I was
going to be fine, I knew the importance of nipping this new fear
in the bud. I can't recall if I asked my higher power for a sign to
rid me of this fear, or whether it was taken note of and surprisingly
delivered to me.

It was early one morning, and I had difficulty sleeping so I
decided to walk down the stairs and watch some television. I heard
two words and then a long pause as I turned on the television set.
I'll never forget those words: *Cancer History.* My new fear has just
been crushed!

When the August 2010 issue of *O* magazine arrived, I once again opened the pages with anticipation. The first page I opened to was an advertisement from the University of Texas Cancer Center. Written on its page is its motto: "Making Cancer History."

Chapter 14

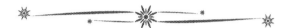

"If we are creating ourselves all the time, then it is never
too late to begin creating the bodies we want instead of
the ones we mistakenly assume we are stuck with."
—Deepak Chopra

Many times, your higher power will present you with unique
spiritual signs, but other times he may present you with reoccurring
symbols that pop up when you least expect them.

I was surprised that it took me awhile to take notice of a
reoccurring symbol that I received throughout my entire cancer
journey—the appearance of butterflies. During my illness, I received
many cards and gifts from my family, friends, and students. Many of
them contained pictures of butterflies. A butterfly would fly by me
whenever I was feeling fear. My son's friends would come over and
draw pictures of butterflies. There was also a picture of a butterfly
on Jann Arden's vision board.

I never clued into the significance of this butterfly symbol until
I received *O* magazine's September 2010 issue. The focus article in
this issue contained illustrations of butterflies and was titled, "Are
You Ready for a Change?" There were pictures of Oprah trying on
various wigs while completely changing her look each time. The
article made the comparison between the changes people undergo

through life and that of a butterfly. If people were to make meaningful changes in their life, then their final product could be as beautiful as a butterfly. This finally made sense as to why I kept receiving this symbol. I was undergoing extreme life changing experiences that could be compared to the various stages of a butterfly's life. The spiritual, emotional, and physical changes I was experiencing were all meant for me to blossom into a butterfly and begin to fly in the direction I wanted to go!

I have often suggested to friends who are experiencing moments of hardship to think of their own symbol and ask their higher power to present them with a symbol—either one they have chosen or a spontaneous one. The joy they experience when they receive it is indescribable, and they are left feeling comforted and their faith restored. Author Pam Grout has written a book titled, *E-Squared*. This book is great for those who wish to begin asking and receiving signs from the universe. It contains nine do-it-yourself energy experiments that *prove* that your thoughts create your reality. "The nine experiments, each of which can be conducted with no money and very little time expenditure, demonstrate that spiritual principles are as dependable as gravity, as consistent as Newton's laws of motion."

I often suggest to my friends to begin asking for signs when they are not experiencing hardship. Ask for them now so that you can become comfortable in receiving them. If you do find yourself in a situation of despair, you are already familiar with the process of asking and receiving, and you can begin to feel comfort immediately. As stated earlier, I was very fortunate that I was able to turn to these signs immediately at the onset of my illness, and thus, I was comforted early. However, regardless of your experience, the universe is just waiting for your call and is eager to jump right in to deliver your message to you!

Chapter 15

"If a man speaks or acts with an evil thought, pain follows
him. If a man speaks or acts with a pure thought, happiness
follows him, like a shadow that never leaves him."
—Gautama Buddha (563-483 BC)

Following the completion of my chemo, I underwent a mastectomy
on my right breast. I was made aware that a new pathology report
would be conducted on the removed breast and lymph nodes.
Knowing that the results will be determining my fate, I continued
focusing on what it was I wanted. Since I wanted a healthy body, I
wrote "good news" on my calendar, specifically on the day I was to
receive my results. I kept referring to my vision board and envisioning
my future in a healthy body. I kept referring to my journal and
reading all the signs I received thus far signaling my survivorship.

While waiting for the results, I was excited to learn that author
Rhonda Bryne's new book, *The Power* had just been released, and
I immediately purchased a copy. The book focuses on the power
we all have to acquire the desires we are seeking including health
by expressing gratitude and love toward ourselves and particularly
to others. The book states, "Give love to others through kindness,
encouragement, gratitude, or any good feeling, and it comes back
to you and multiplies itself, bringing love to every other area of

your life, including your health, money, happiness, and career. Give negativity to others, through criticism, anger, impatience or any bad feeling and you will receive that negativity back—guaranteed! And as the negativity comes back, it multiplies itself, attracting more negativity, which affects the rest of your life."

In essence, your feelings that you give toward others is like a boomerang! What you give out is what you receive back. I knew that I had to change my negative feelings toward one specific individual, but I was not successful because I thought I had to give out feelings of love. To be quite honest, I didn't find any particular trait about this person that was worthy of love, and as a result, I continued to foster negative thoughts. Little did I know that those negative thoughts were directed right back at me, affecting every part of my life including my health.

I remembered the exhilarating feeling I experienced throughout my entire body when I read a passage in *The Power* that stated, "Part of the gift of life is that you are given all kinds of people, so you can choose what you love in those people and turn away from what you don't love. You are not meant to manufacture love for qualities in a person you don't love, but simply to turn away without giving them any feeling."

After several years of struggling to come to peace with this person, I finally received my answer! Simply refuse to give *any* thoughts to this person. If you can't find any qualities to love about a person, and you realize that you must not give out *any* negative thoughts, then simply don't think any thoughts at all! I knew I could this! Whenever a negative thought about this person would appear in my mind, I would say, "Stop" to myself and visualize myself closing a curtain over the face of the person, stopping all thoughts from emerging. Gradually through practicing this strategy, I eventually found myself not only free from thinking any negative thoughts toward this person but all thoughts. I rarely even thought of this person anymore!

Who would have realized that a simple training of the mind could result in finally having peace with my thoughts? How happy was I to know that by simply controlling my mind to stop thinking negative thoughts, I was aiding my body in healing both spiritually and physically!

Chapter 16

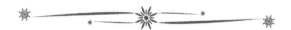

"To believe in the thing you can see and touch is no belief at all; but to believe in the unseen is a triumph and a blessing."
—Abraham Lincoln (1809–1865)

Just as I was informed of my cancer diagnosis through Oprah's May 2010 issue of *O* magazine, it was through the October 2010 issue that I was informed of my fate as well!

On that particular night, my husband and I decided to go Christmas shopping for our son. While waiting in line to purchase the toys we selected, I noticed the October issue of *O* magazine at the checkout counter. I couldn't help but feel the urgent need to purchase it, despite the fact that I would be receiving my issue any day. I just had my surgery and I was waiting for my pathology report. Knowing that each monthly magazine issue had delivered me with articles that related to my unique experiences, I couldn't help but wonder what this issue contained.

I decided to purchase it. On our way home, we stopped at a fast food restaurant. My husband went in to purchase the food while I waited in the car. I instantly pulled out the magazine. I couldn't wait any longer. The first article I opened sent me into a state of crazy emotions, and I began crying hysterically. At this point my husband returned and was concerned about what he was seeing. I handed him the article. The article was titled, "I'm a Cancer Survivor." The article featured three breast cancer survivors. I felt my whole body let loose. I wanted to lie down in the back seat because I found it difficult keeping my body in an upward position. My body was experiencing this huge sigh of relief!

God wanted to be the first one to share the good news with me. He knew I would listen just as I did in the previous issues. He also decided to share one more article with me. He wanted to make sure I was clear about how my new state came about. Once I stopped crying, I turned to an article titled, "The Law of Attraction." I knew immediately that by following the principles behind the law of attraction, such as visualizing, asking, believing, and releasing negativity and fear-based thinking, the universe had responded.

Chapter 17

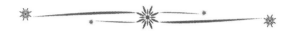

"I accept perfect health as the natural state of my being.
I now consciously release any mental patterns within
me that could express as disease in any way. Perfect
health is my Divine right, and I claim it now."

—Louise Hay

Early in November of 2010, I received the results of my pathology report from my doctor. When they analysed the breast tissue, only 0.7 millimetres of cancer remained from a tumor size of 8 centimeters by 9 centimeters. My doctor expressed her surprise at the unlikelihood of this happening. I remembered sitting there long after the doctor left the room and not feeling the least bit surprised. I was clearly elated but not shocked. I finally witnessed the connection between the mind and body. When the mind is at peace, the body is as well! I also understood how a simple process of asking for your desire, visualizing your goal, releasing the fear and doubt about its attainment, and finally being in a state of love can bring your desire into being. By releasing negative thought patterns and substituting them with loving thoughts that are always directed in the direction you want to go, you can experience your dreams no matter how big they are.

I continued sitting there in the doctor's office and feeling so full of gratitude. I was extremely grateful that God was able to send forth spiritual signs in a manner that allowed me to figure out what I needed to do to heal. I was also grateful that I was open to receiving and believing in its message.

I need to reinforce the fact that *I am not special*! The signs given to me are given to anyone who is open to receiving them. The specific messages are ideas he wants everyone to know in order to heal themselves from any ailment. In God's eyes, *we are already healed*! It is up to us to tap into the power He has already given us the day we were born. My messages I received are universal messages for *everyone* who has a vision to achieve their desires including health, abundance, relationships and so forth.

I am eternally grateful that I am able to share what messages were given to me from God, the universe, or our higher power to share with others. I was fortunate I was in tune to these signs, but for the majority of people who aren't, please follow the messages that I was receptive to receiving; the very least, *believe in the intention of these messages for everyone*!

Chapter 18

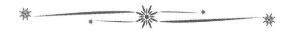

"Miracles are God's way of remaining anonymous."
—Author unknown

Within the next few weeks following my joyous news, I occasionally found myself questioning what truly caused the tumor to essentially disappear. In stillness, I always knew my answer, but my ego allowed me to doubt my knowingness. Could it really be the chemotherapy alone that shrunk the huge tumor to nothingness? That's the impression I was getting from others. If this was the case, then why aren't other people's tumors disappearing as well? As I found myself arguing with my ego about my true source of healing, the December 2010 issue of *O* magazine arrived. My ego could finally take a back seat to this debate. This would be the final issue I received during my cancer journey; its message didn't get any better than this: "Miracles All Around Us." This was the magazine's special feature of the month. "Witness Earth's most staggering natural wonders, discover mysteries that science can't solve and meet a few ordinary people whose extraordinary experiences defy explanation. Martha Beck shares the secret to finding miracles where you least expect them."

Yes, I did indeed receive a miracle from God, and for this I am eternally grateful. However, once again, *I am not special*! I experienced a miracle, however, it wasn't a special gift chosen solely for me.

Regardless of your past experiences and beliefs, you are worthy of a miracle. God doesn't select a few to be chosen and disregard the rest. As stated in *A Course of Miracles*, "What order can there be in miracles, unless someone deserves to suffer more and others less? And is this justice to the wholly innocent? A miracle *is* justice. It is not a special gift to some, to be withheld from others as less worthy, more condemned, and thus apart from healing. Where is salvation's justice if some errors are unforgivable and warrant vengeance in place of healing and return of peace? *Everyone* is equally entitled to His gift of healing and deliverance and peace. Its offering is universal, and it teaches but one message: *What is God's belongs to everyone, and is his due.*"

"Miracles do not happen in contradiction to nature, but
only in contradiction to what is known in nature."
—St. Augustine (Latin Philosopher and Theologian)

Chapter 19

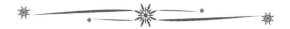

"What seems to us bitter trials are often blessings in disguise."
—Oscar Wilde

As I reflect back on my cancer journey, I now have more clarity as to how I could experience true happiness at a time where the outcome of my life was greatly questionable.

First, I never regarded cancer as a battle I needed to "fight against." Logically, if you choose to fight against anything, you have a 50 percent chance of losing, and that's a high risk for anyone to take on. Furthermore, when you fight against anything, including disease, you are exerting negative energy toward the subject, and anytime you put out negativity, you are certain to receive it back, regardless of your intention.

I didn't regard cancer as an evil substance in my body that I wanted to attack despite the fact I wanted it gone. Somehow, by knowing intuitively and instantly that my dysfunctional thoughts contributed to the onset of this disease, I regarded cancer as a means to help me repair my dysfunctional thoughts so that I could begin to enjoy life once again! As spiritual leader and author Wayne Dyer wrote in his book, *Real Magic*, when faced with a health ailment, he suggests asking, "*What do I have to learn from this disease, or this lack of health?* What is the lesson here? Then begin to apply your new awareness about the power of your mind to alter that debilitating state you have previously accepted as your destiny."

I knew immediately I had many lessons to learn. I didn't realize at that first moment what my lessons were, but I knew I had them, and I was determined to figure out what they were and come to peace with them. Cancer allowed me to go deep within and somehow *fix* what was broken inside of me. *Cancer was simply a tool used to help me get happy again!* Somewhere down the road, I lost my direction, and cancer helped me to get back on track again. I was *happy with cancer* because *I embraced its purpose!* Each morning to this day, I wake up thanking the universe for this most amazing life-changing cancer experience!

Also, I somehow intuitively felt that I needed to *believe* I was going to survive. Too often we talk ourselves out of believing we can achieve what we desire, especially when it comes to our health. We allow doctor's doubts, our own doubts, fears, and the discouraging things people say to us to convince us we can't achieve what we want. I never once asked my doctor's opinion as to my chances of surviving this disease with a tumor size as large as it was. What would be the purpose other than trying to control that voice that would be screaming in my head each day? I still have no idea what my first pathology report stated. I still have it, but I never wished for its explanation. I knew it wasn't promising, but I consciously chose not to go there. I had only one vision, and I wasn't going to let anyone or anything get in the way of achieving it. Somehow, whenever I became real still, I would become comforted with the knowingness that deep down within me, *my creator does not want me to die.* I challenge anyone with a serious health ailment to get still and feel this knowingness as well!

I was also happy and fortunate that the closest people in my life never focused on my illness. My husband, mother, closest friends, and family members were able to allow me to continue on with my life as if I never received a cancer diagnosis. This was so important because since I was only focused on healing and visioning my life as disease free, then I needed to be around those who allowed me to experience this. Those closest to me never displayed their fears to me, which is what I needed. Since I was working on letting go of my fears, I knew I needed to be around people who did not let their fear have an impact on me. As people began hearing about my illness, their reaction determined whether they were going to be a presence in my life or not. Any fear-based statements or energy from people clearly signaled to me that I needed distance from them. I quickly learned that those who expressed fear-based comments to me ultimately were those who were experiencing their own personal fears about disease. Surrounding myself only with people who didn't regard me as a cancer patient but my true self was truly a gift from above.

Finally, it was my ability to release the fear, resistance, and anger that was within me to not only heal my body but feel happy and joyful during the process as well. Whether someone is experiencing cancer or any other health ailment, it is important to *be still* and *look inward* for true causes. It is through this first step of inward reflection that healing begins and miracles transpire!

About the Author

Linda Ranalli-Marr is an author, elementary school teacher, wife, and mother. She was inspired to write this book to help others to *look inward* for true causes of disease and utilize their inner knowingness and power to heal themselves. Linda lives in Welland, Ontario, with her family.

Printed in the United States
By Bookmasters